Just like the Ocean

a yoga journey for parent and baby

written by Emily Foster Williams
illustrated by Sabdo Purnomo

For Eleanor & June.

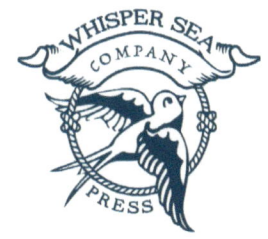

My sweet little baby,
Let's take time today,
We can set aside our cares
And go tiptoe away,

I'll tell you a story
About you and me,
The story starts here
At the edge of the sea.

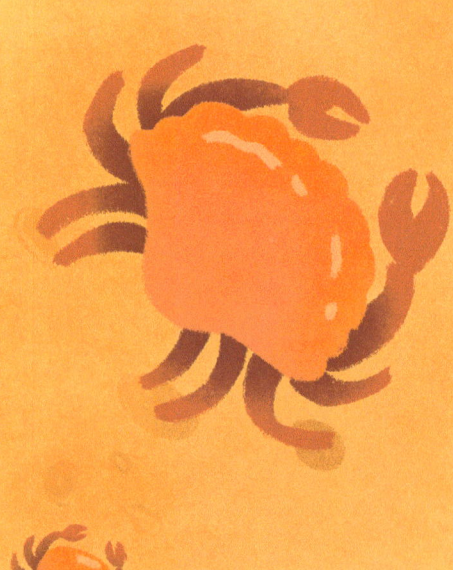

This story provides gentle movement for new mothers or fathers and most babies ages 6 weeks and up. Follow along with the story and the coordinating movements by matching the story to the numbered yoga postures.

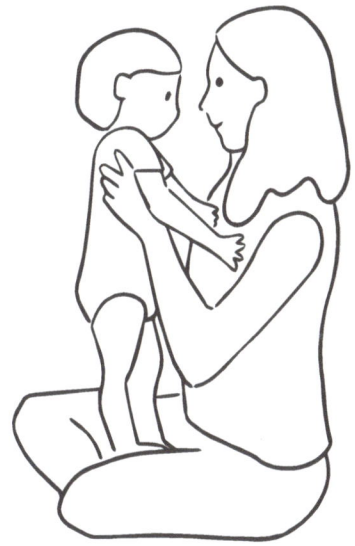

1 On the floor, sitting comfortably, take time to connect with your baby face to face.

Yogi Says ★

Try relaxing your facial muscles during your yoga practice. Now, doesn't that feel nice?

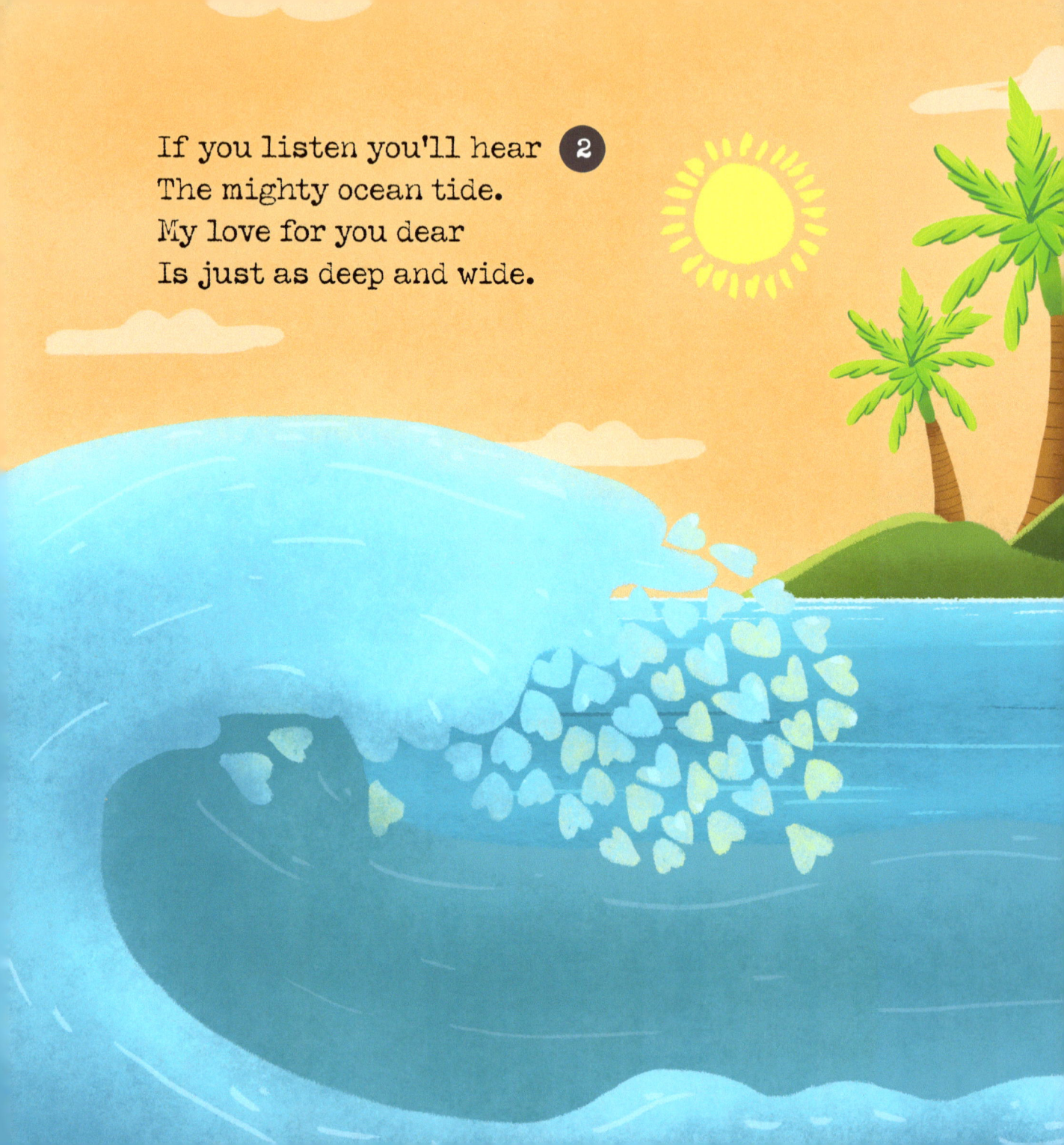

If you listen you'll hear
The mighty ocean tide.
My love for you dear
Is just as deep and wide.

② Ujjayi Breathing

With baby on lap, slowly and deeply breathe through your nose, extending your exhale as long as you can and letting the air swirl in the back of your throat. This breath continues throughout your yoga practice.

Gently sway side to side on your "sit" bones, imitating the rhythm of the ocean.

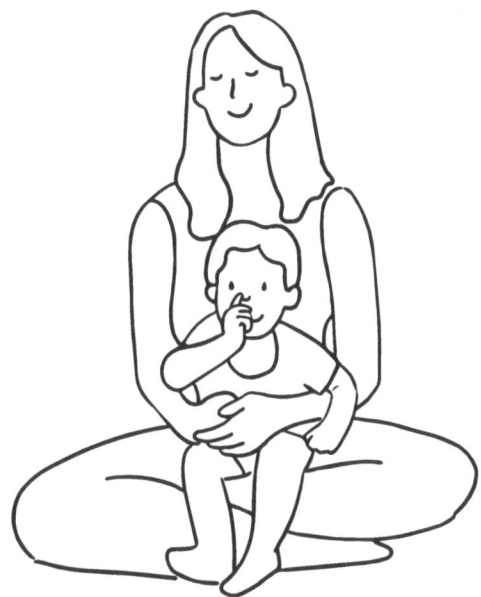

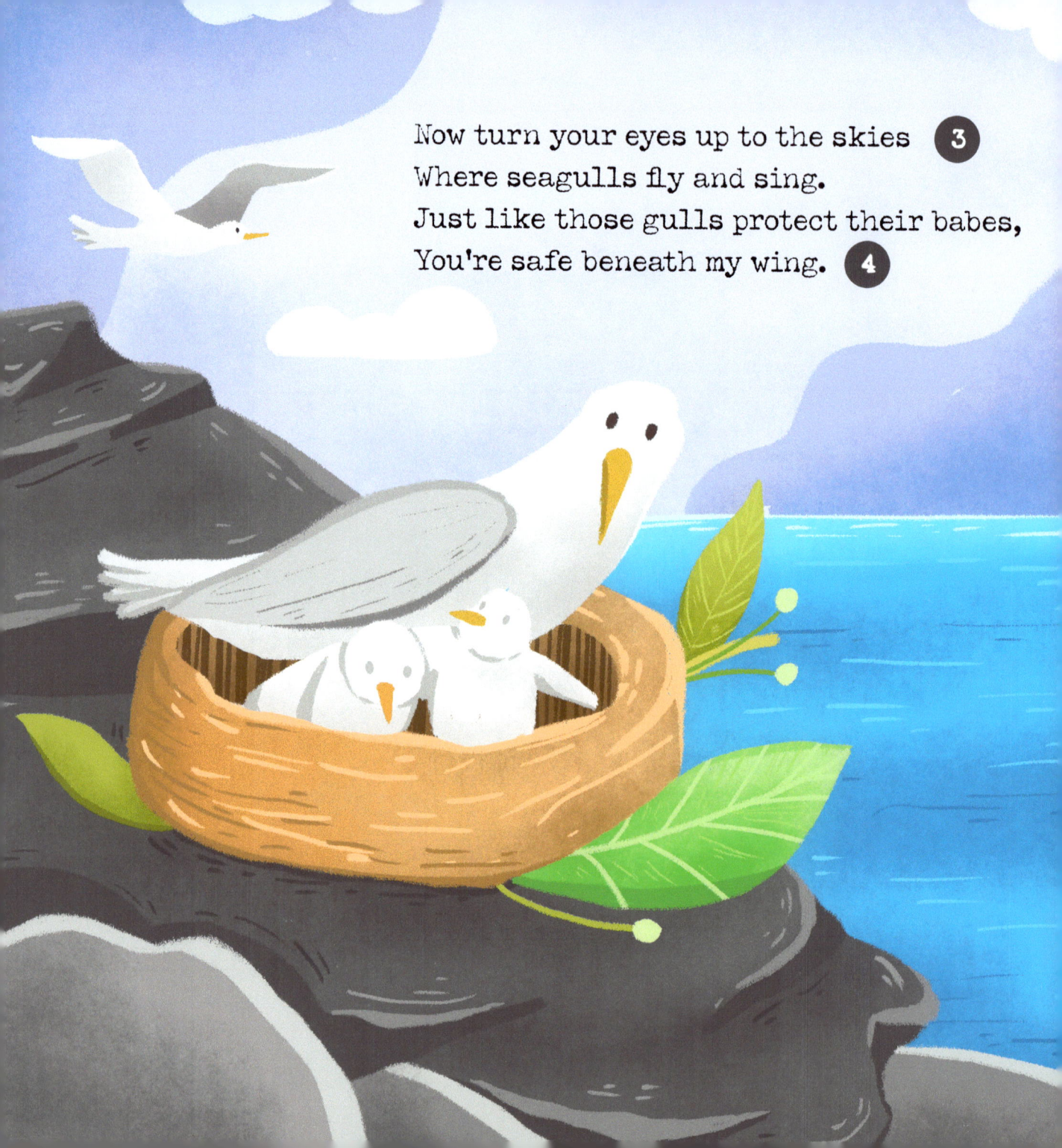

Now turn your eyes up to the skies ③
Where seagulls fly and sing.
Just like those gulls protect their babes,
You're safe beneath my wing. ④

3. Neck Stretch

Gently roll your head in circles, taking extra time to go over sore or stiff spots. Older babies will have fun trying this, too!

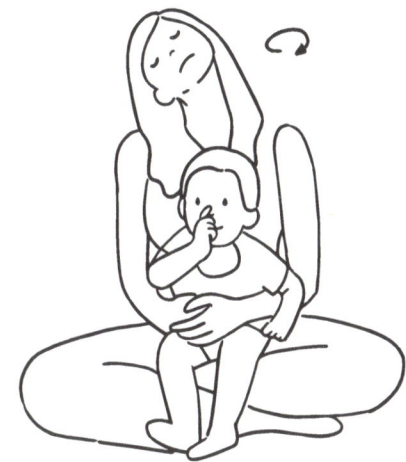

4. Seated Side-Stretch

Cradling your baby, extend one arm over your head and stretch toward the opposite wall. With each inhale, stretch out longer; with each exhale, lower toward the floor. Stop when your sit bones begin to lift off the floor. Feel the stretch in your back, side, and arm. Feel your shoulders relax as you bend over. Ahhh …

Repeat opposite side.

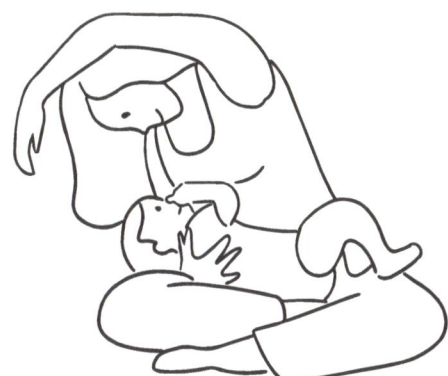

Yogi Says ⭐

Try timing your movements with your breath. Take your time, there's no rush.

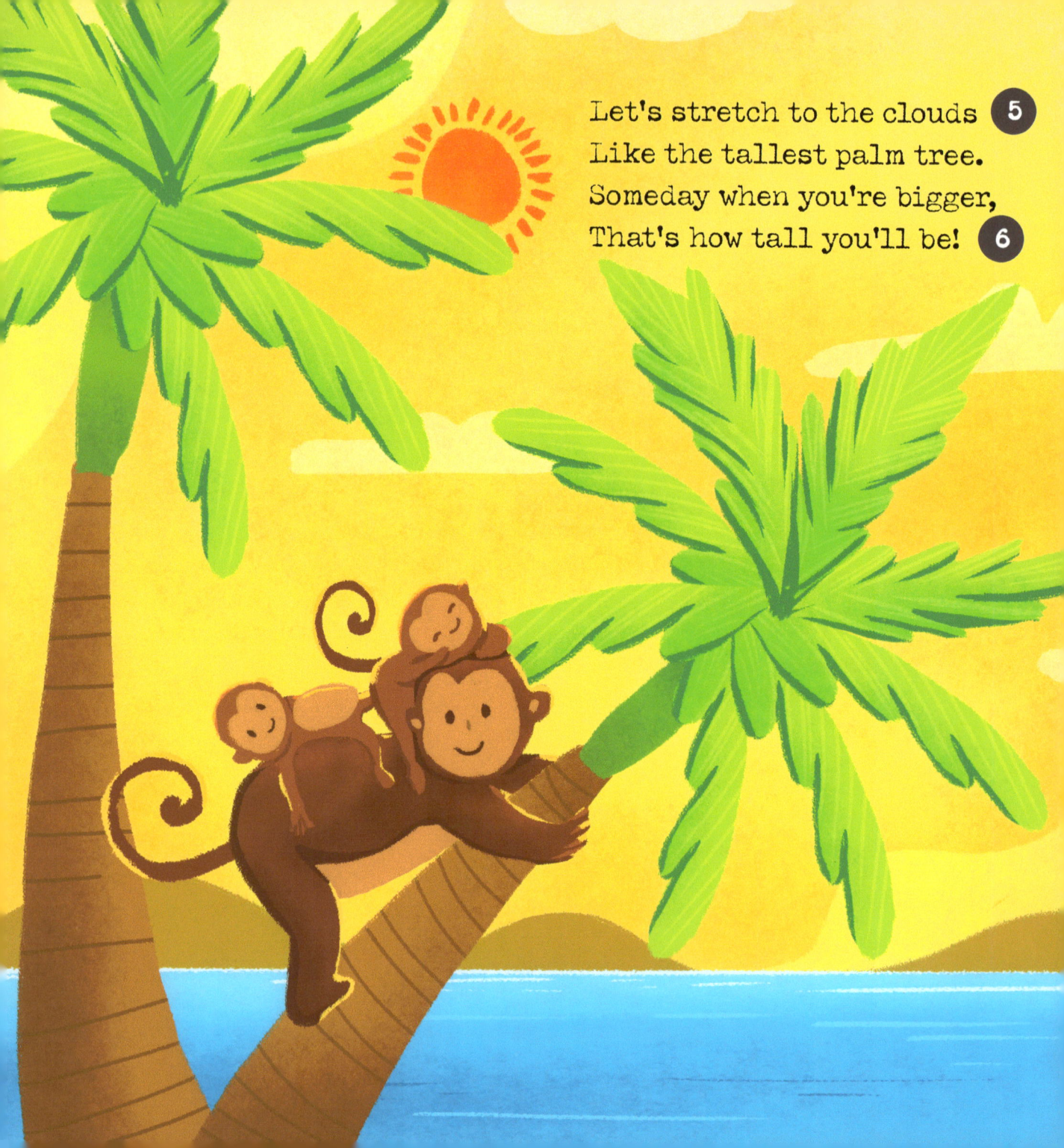

Let's stretch to the clouds
Like the tallest palm tree.
Someday when you're bigger,
That's how tall you'll be!

5 Cowface Pose

Extend one hand high into the air, then reach behind your head to grasp the opposite hand, palms together. If you can't do this, use your other hand to pull on the elbow pointed at the ceiling.

Repeat opposite side.

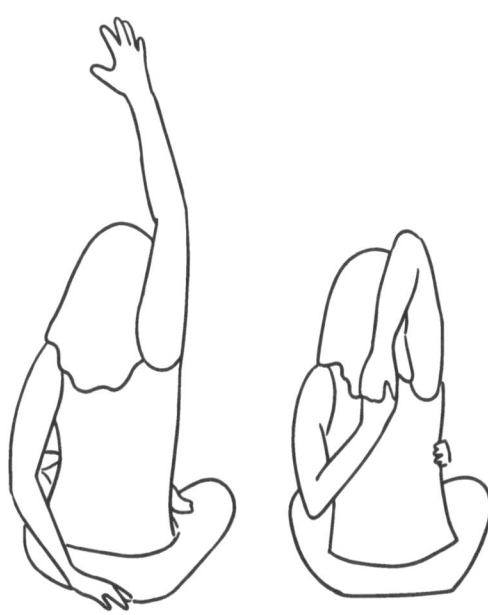

6 Chest Opener

With legs folded beneath you, place one hand behind you towards the center of your body. Drop your head back, allowing your arm to support your weight.

Repeat opposite side.

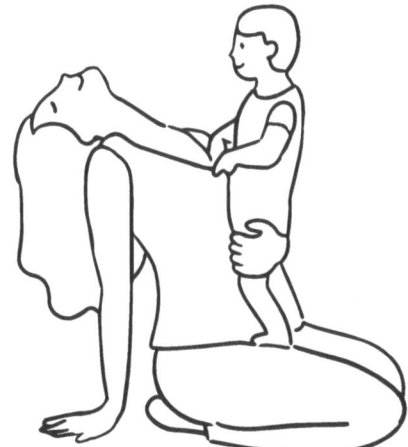

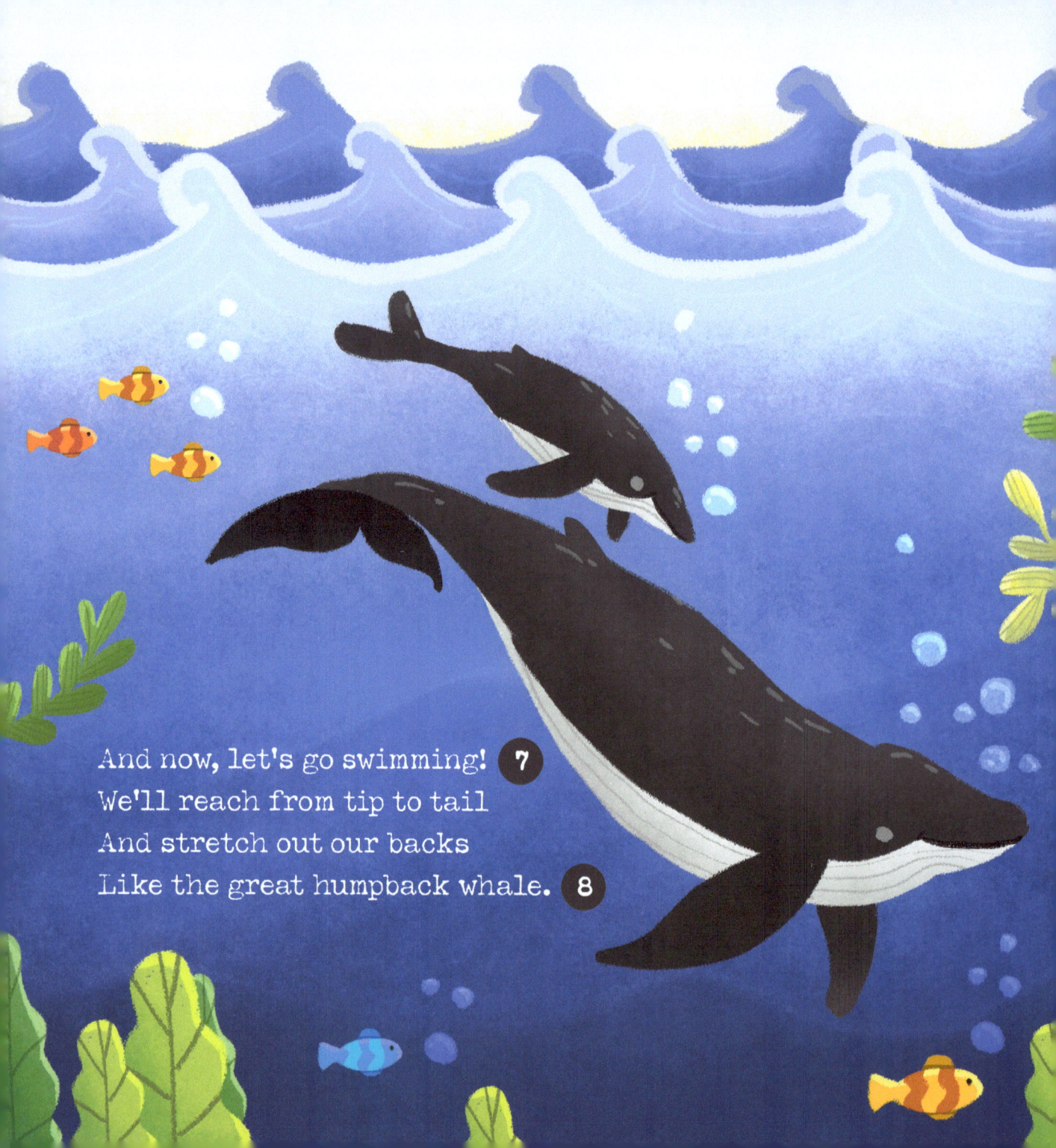

And now, let's go swimming! 7
We'll reach from tip to tail
And stretch out our backs
Like the great humpback whale. 8

7. Table Pose Extensions

Starting with your hands under your shoulders and knees under your hips, stretch one arm and your opposite leg away from your body, parallel to the floor. Tickle your baby!

Repeat opposite side.

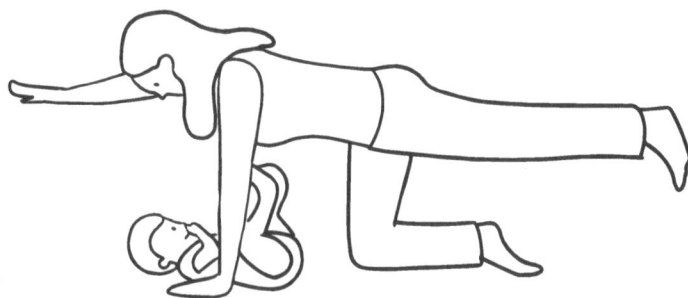

8. Cat & Cow Pose

Round out your back like a cat, rolling your shoulders toward your ears.

Then, let your back drop towards the floor like a cow, pointing your sit bones toward the ceiling.

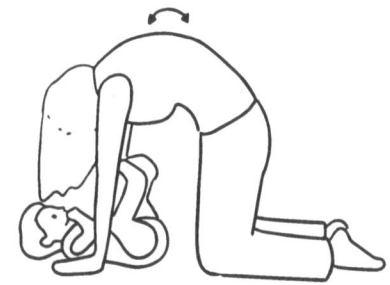

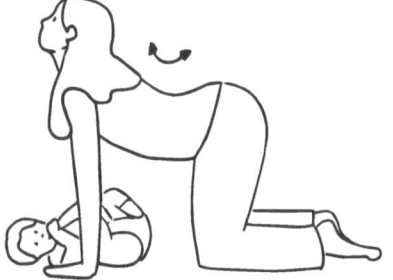

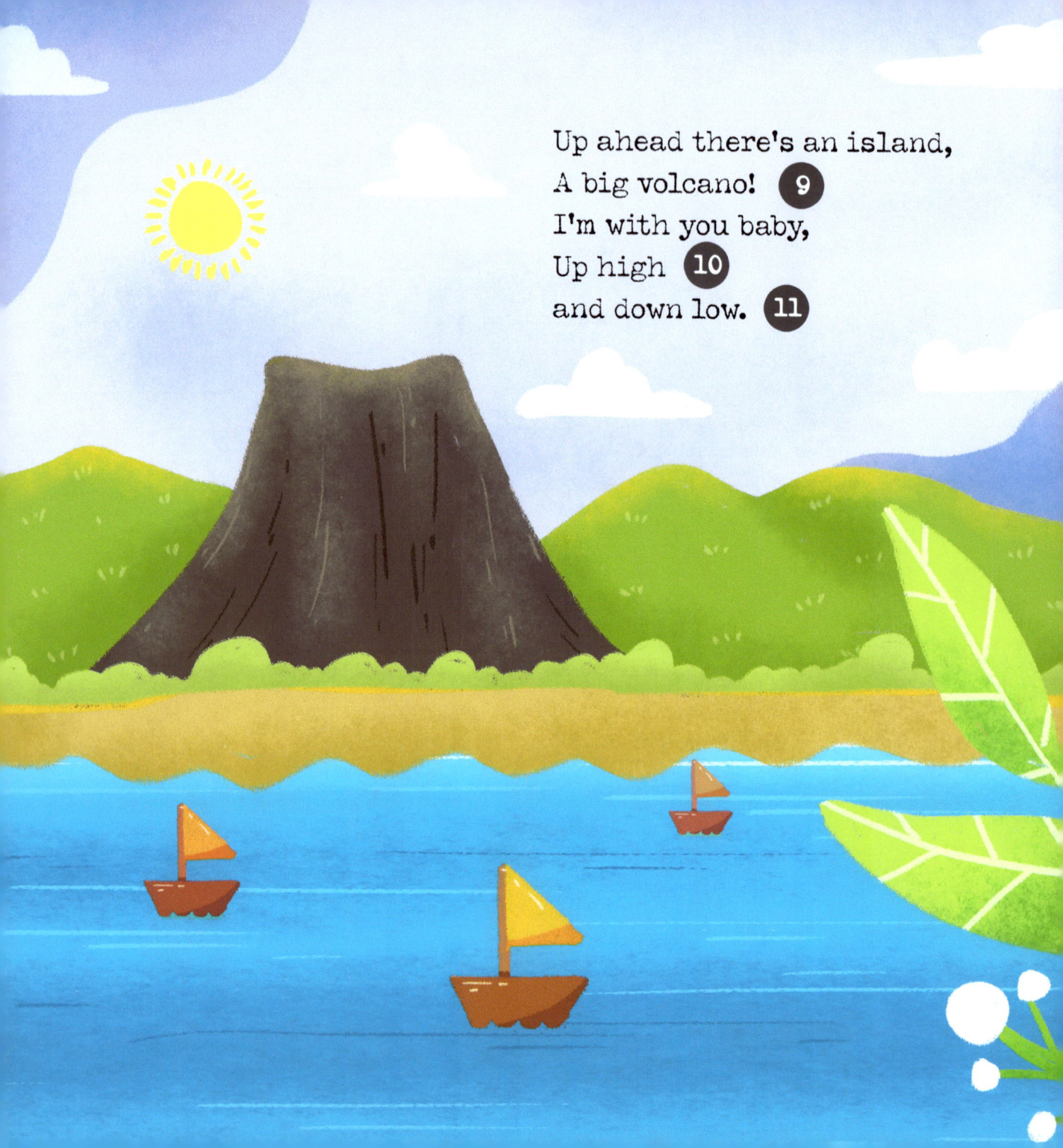

Up ahead there's an island,
A big volcano!
I'm with you baby,
Up high
and down low.

9. Downward Facing Dog

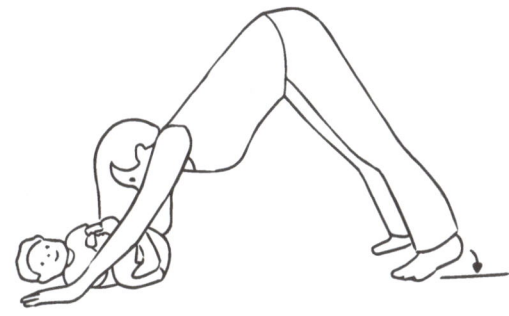

With feet shoulder-width apart, raise your hips high into the air, pointing your sit bones to the ceiling. Pull most of your weight onto your legs by stretching your back and straightening your arms. Work on slowly straightening your legs and getting your heels to touch the floor.

10. Upward Facing Dog

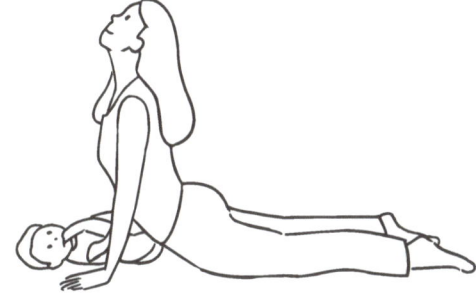

Drop your body into a push-up position or Plank Pose, then lower hips close to the floor and raise your chest into the air. Work on keeping your hips off the ground and your shoulders down and back to open your chest.

11. Child's Pose

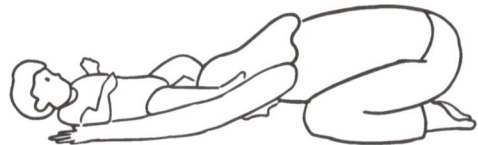

Push your body back over your knees, sitting on your heels to rest for a moment. It may feel more comfortable to widen your knees. Older babies love to do this pose with you!

Yogi Says

Repeat these three poses several times for an aerobic workout.

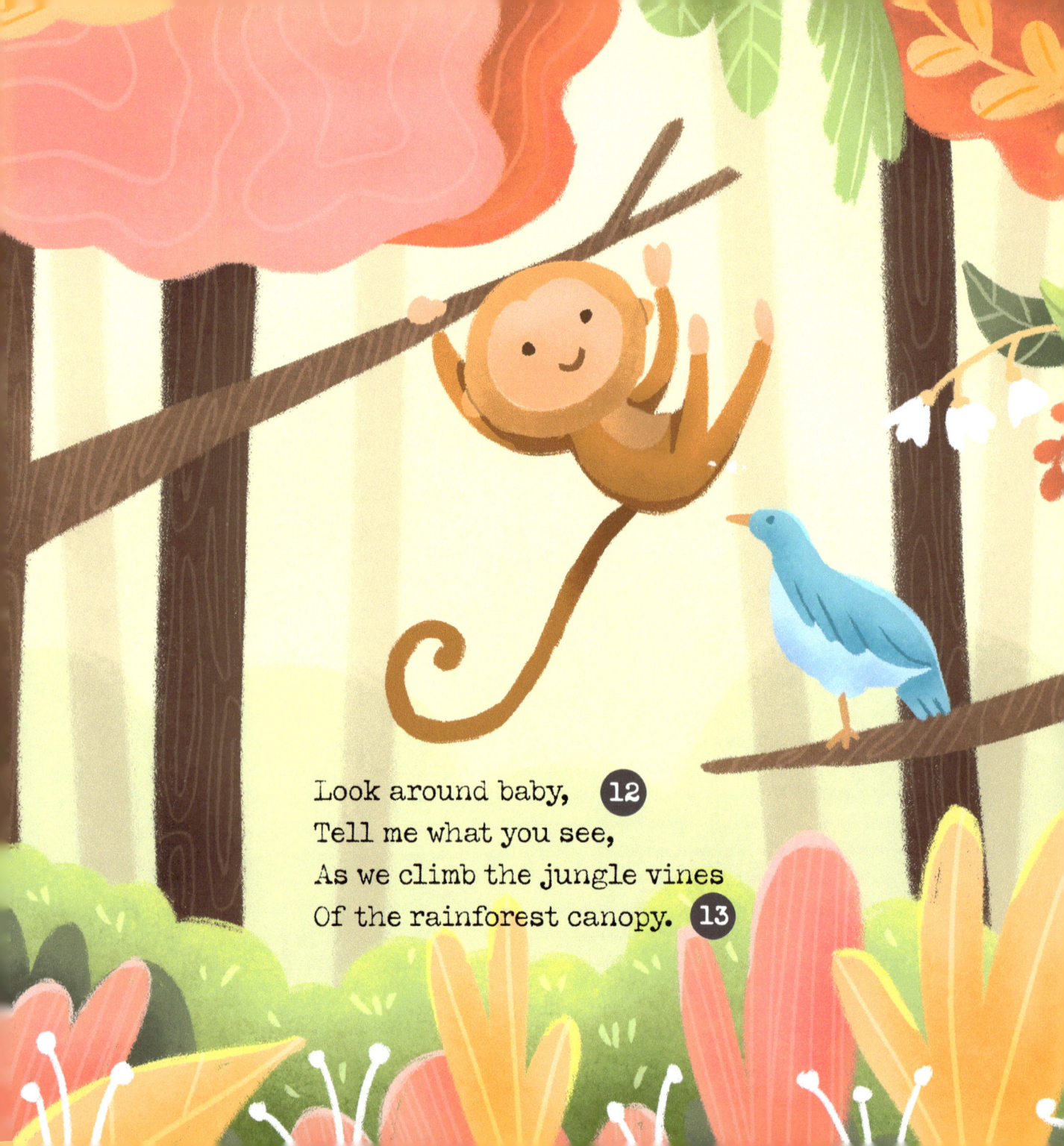

12 Mountain Pose

With parallel feet shoulder-width apart, stand up tall; straightening your spine, drawing your shoulders down and back, drawing your abdomen upward and in, rooting your soles into the ground.

Talk to your baby about what he or she sees.

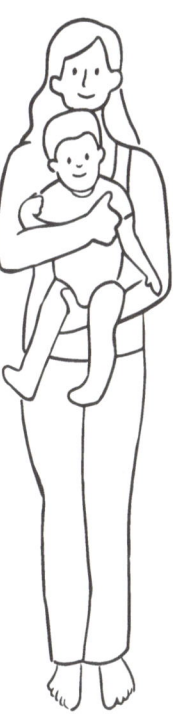

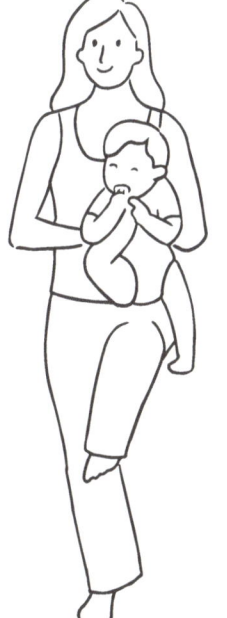

13 Tree Pose

Slowly raise one knee, sliding the bottom of your foot up the opposite leg. Balance here for a moment, with baby sitting on your thigh.

Repeat opposite leg.

Yogi Says

Don't worry if you can't get the pose just right. Yoga takes a lifetime to perfect.

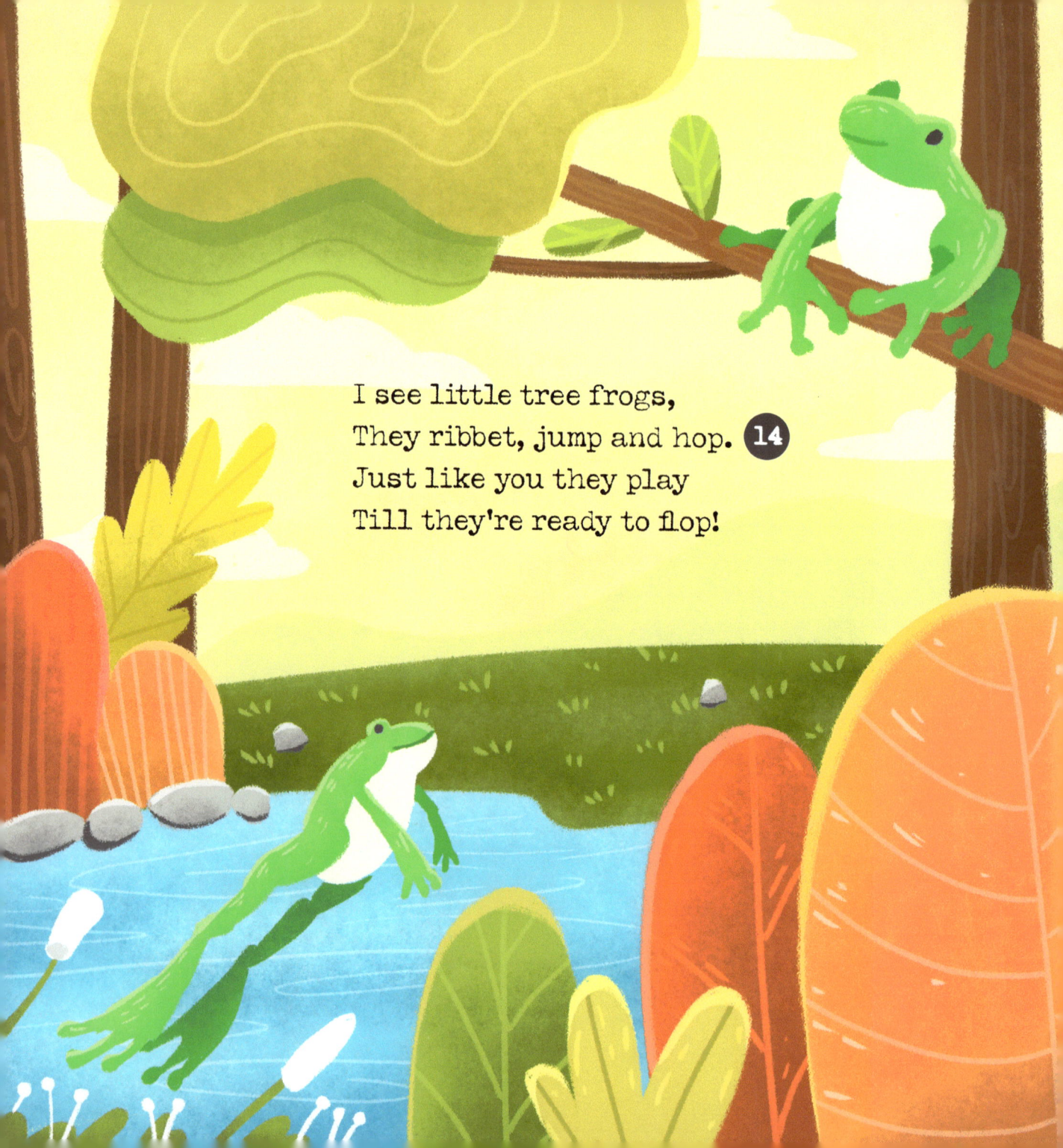

I see little tree frogs,
They ribbet, jump and hop.
Just like you they play
Till they're ready to flop!

14 Frog Squats

With feet a little wider than hip-width apart, slowly squat down until your sit bones nearly reach the floor. Add Kegel exercises to aid in birthing recovery.

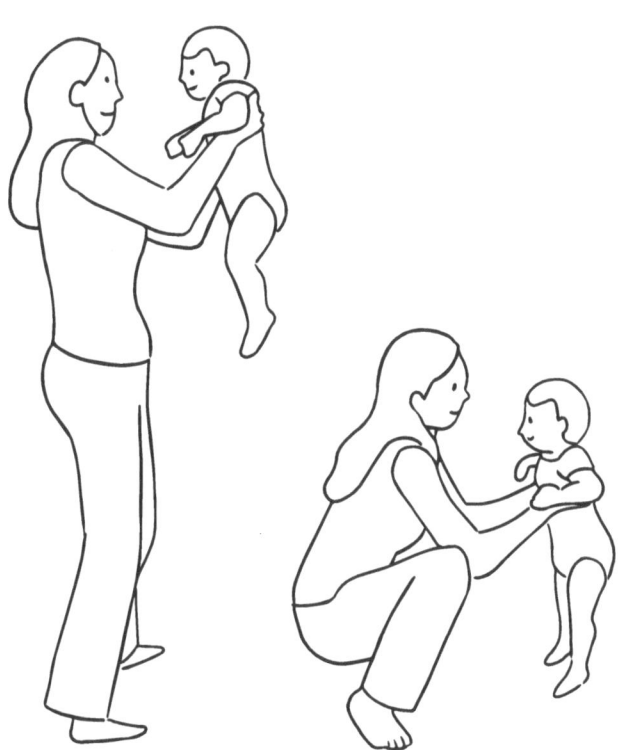

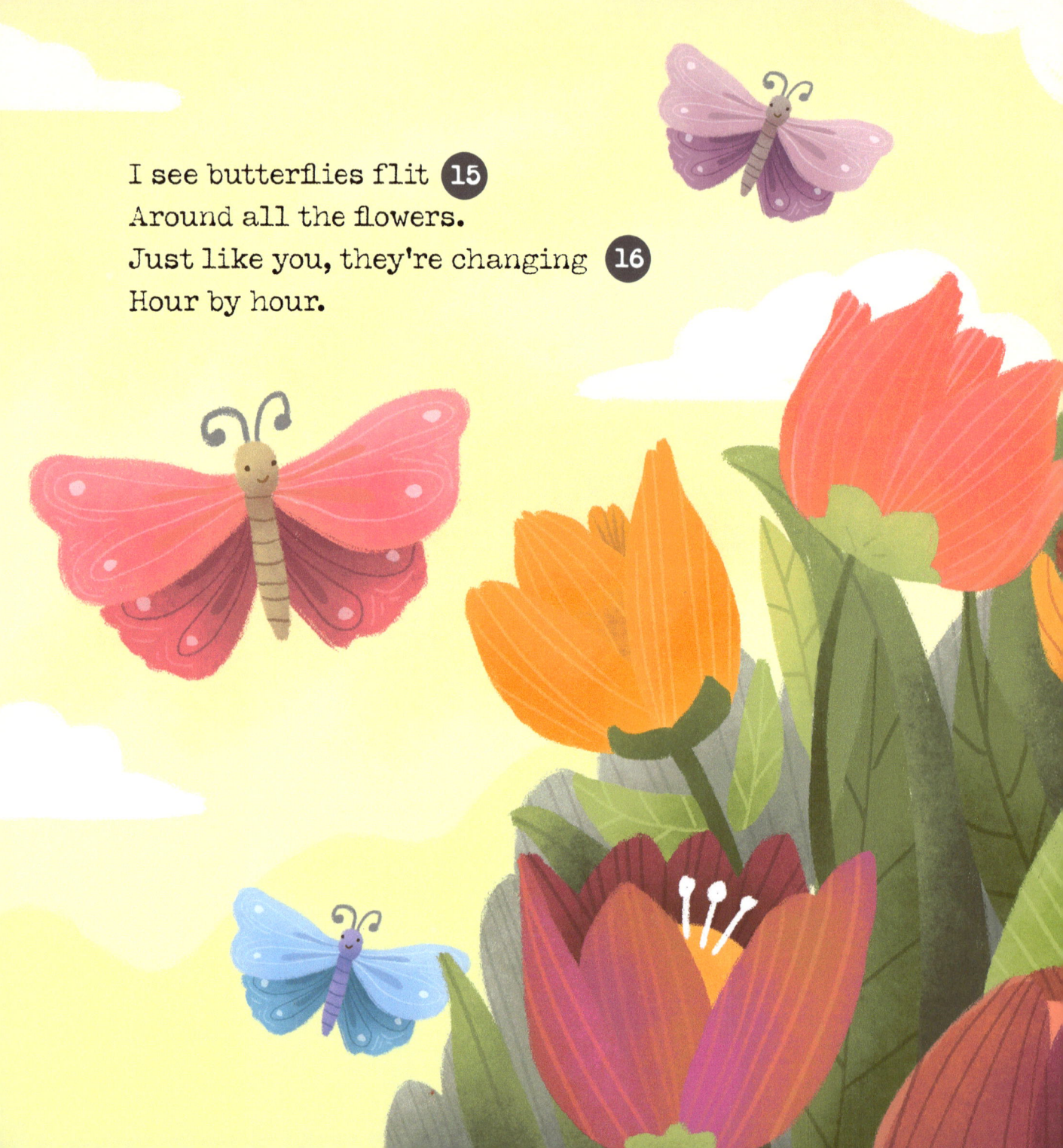

I see butterflies flit 15
Around all the flowers.
Just like you, they're changing 16
Hour by hour.

15. Butterfly Pose

Sitting on the floor, bring your feet together close to your body. Relax your legs toward the floor.

Your baby might enjoy tummy time, or doing the pose along with you.

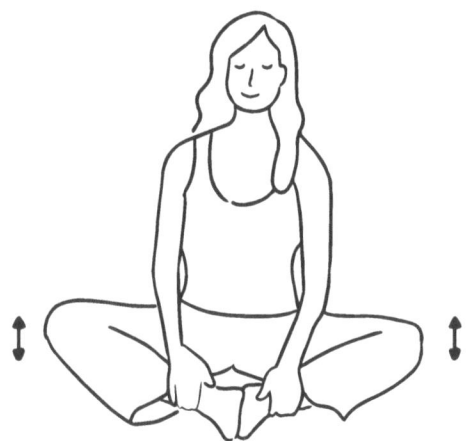

16. Seated Twist

With legs in front of you, place one foot outside the opposite knee. Turn away from your bent leg, gently stretching your back while your baby stands. Hold for several breaths before twisting toward your leg, bringing your baby with you.

Repeat opposite side.

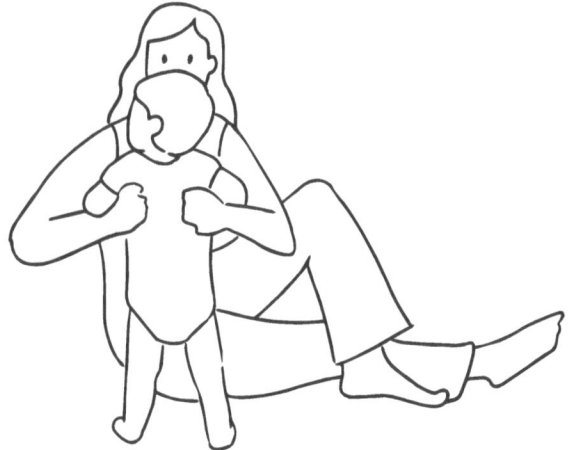

Let's hop in a boat now 17
And sail our way home.
Just like Captain and First Mate,
We'll never be alone.

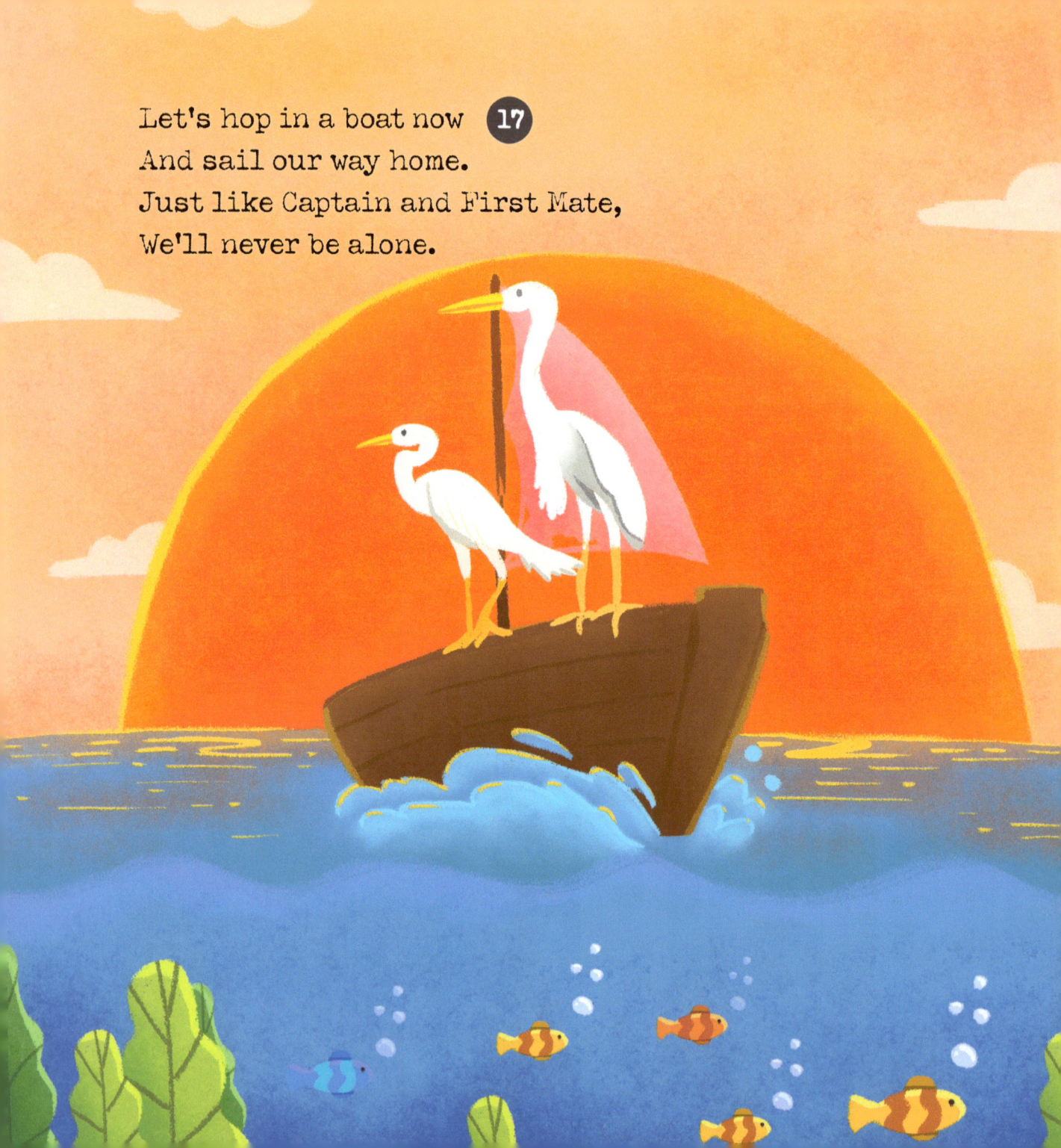

17 Boat Pose

Sit with your knees bent, and your baby laying on your thighs. Then, slowly lean back as you raise your feet into the air. Keep your arms and legs parallel to the ground and your back straight. Balance here for a moment.

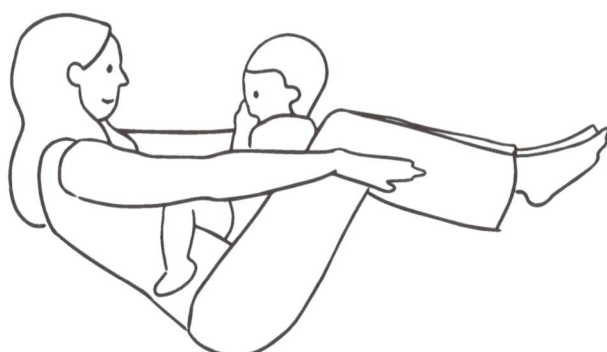

Yogi Says

This is a great pose for regaining abdominal muscle tone after pregnancy. Just first make sure that your doctor or midwife says you're ready for this exercise.

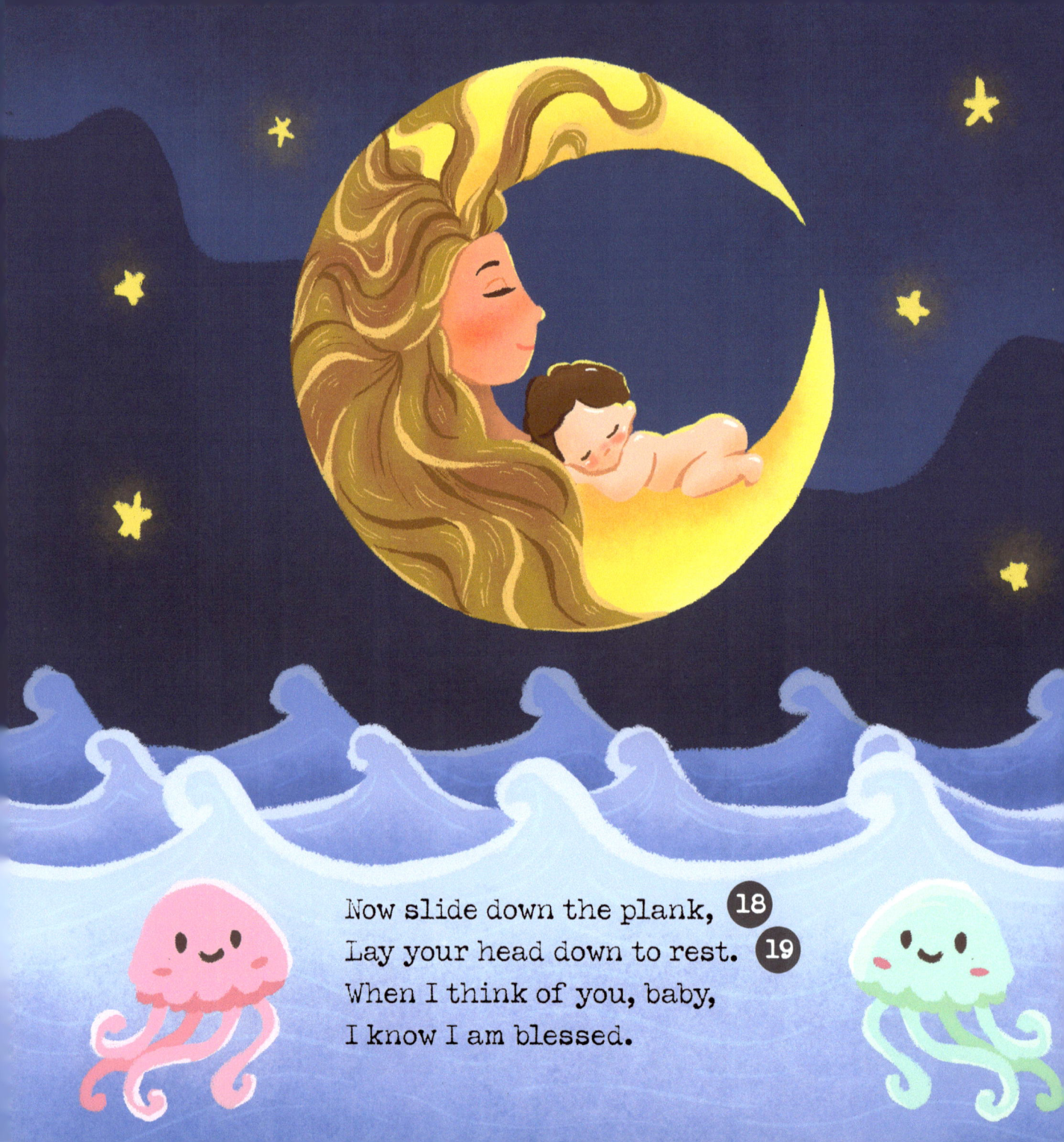

Now slide down the plank, **18**
Lay your head down to rest. **19**
When I think of you, baby,
I know I am blessed.

18 Bridge Pose

From Boat Pose, lower your back to the floor and place your feet under your knees. Lift your hips into the air. Lengthen your spine, keeping your collarbone away form your ears.

Try massaging your baby's feet and legs.

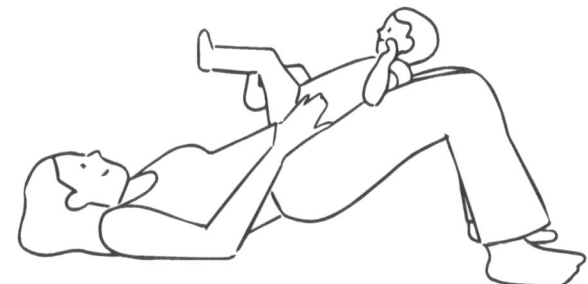

19 Resting Pose

Lie flat on your back, heart-to-heart with your baby. Close your eyes and relax your breathing, allowing your body to rest and recover from your yoga practice.

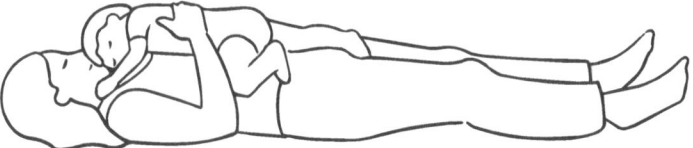

First Whisper Sea Company Press Edition 2025

Text copyright ©2020 by Emily Foster Williams

Illustrations by Sabdo Purnomo copyright ©Emily Foster Williams

WHISPER SEA Cº | PRESS

An imprint of Whisper Sea Company, LLC
St. Augustine, FL 32080

All rights reserved, including the right of reproduction in whole or in part in any form or by any means, except for the inclusion in a review or retailer marketing.

For information about this title contact the publisher:
Whisper Sea Company Press | wscstudio@outlook.com

Library of Congress Control Number: 2020909425

ISBN:
Hardcover: 978-1-7333829-2-2 | EPUB: 978-1-7333829-3-9

www.ingramcontent.com/pod-product-compliance
Lightning Source LLC
Chambersburg PA
CBHW041408160426
42811CB00103B/1550